Anti-Inflammatory Cookbook

Salads and Side dish Recipes for your everyday meals

Natalie Worley

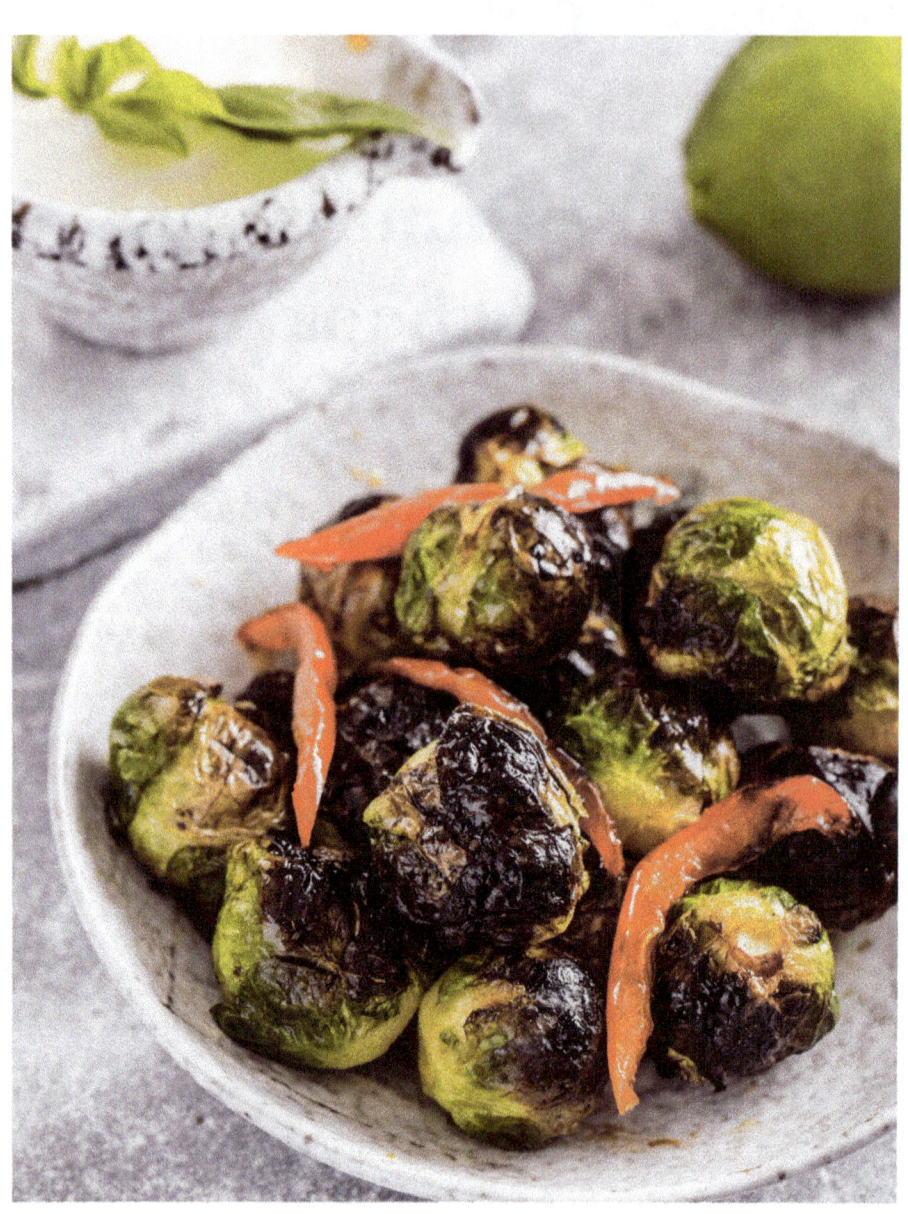

© copyright 2021 – all rights reserved.

the content contained within this book may not be reproduced, duplicated or transmitted without direct written permission from the author or the publisher.

under no circumstances will any blame or legal responsibility be held against the publisher, or author, for any damages, reparation, or monetary loss due to the information contained within this book. either directly or indirectly.

legal notice:

this book is copyright protected. this book is only for personal use. you cannot amend, distribute, sell, use, quote or paraphrase any part, or the content within this book, without the consent of the author or publisher.

disclaimer notice:

please note the information contained within this document is for educational and entertainment purposes only. all effort has been executed to present accurate, up to date, and reliable, complete information. no warranties of any kind are declared or implied. readers acknowledge that the author is not engaging in the rendering of legal, financial, medical or professional advice. the content within this book has been derived from various sources. please consult a licensed professional before attempting any techniques outlined in this book.

by reading this document, the reader agrees that under no circumstances is the author responsible for any losses, direct or indirect, which are incurred as a result of the use of information contained within this document, including, but not limited to, — errors, omissions, or inaccuracies.

Table of Contents

- LIME BRUSSELS SPROUTS 6
- CABBAGE BOWL 8
- PARMESAN ASPARAGUS 10
- COCONUT QUINOA 11
- ROSEMARY BLACK BEANS 12
- OREGANO GREEN BEANS 13
- YAM MASH 16
- SOFT PEAS 17
- MUSHROOM STEW 19
- CHEESY BROCCOLI 21
- GLAZED BROCCOLI 23
- CINNAMON ASPARAGUS 25
- SPICY CUCUMBERS 27
- SPRING SALAD 29
- TENDER QUINOA 32
- CHICKPEAS BOWL 33
- BEANS MASH 35
- SPIRALIZED CARROT 37
- CLASSIC BARLEY 39
- BAKED MANGO 40
- EASY CABBAGE SLAW 41
- APPLE SALAD 44
- AVOCADO MASH 45
- BAKE ENDIVES 47
- ARUGULA BOWL 48
- POTATO MASH 49
- CREAMY SWEET POTATO MASH 51
- GINGERED CAULIFLOWER RICE 53
- SPICY CAULIFLOWER RICE 55
- SIMPLE BROWN RICE 58

SPICY QUINOA	60
QUINOA WITH APRICOTS	62
EASY ZUCCHINI SLAW	64
BROC N' CHEESE	65
GREEK AVGOLEMONO SOUP	68
ITALIAN ZUPPA DI POMODORO	70
EASY ZUCCHINI CROQUETS	73
PORK AND CHEESE STUFFED PEPPERS	75
STEWED CABBAGE WITH GOAN CHORIZO SAUSAGE	78
CAULIFLOWER AND HAM CASSEROLE	80
STUFFED SPAGHETTI SQUASH	82
SPICY AND WARM COLESLAW	84
EASY MEDITERRANEAN CROQUETTES	87
TUSCAN ASPARAGUS WITH CHEESE	89
BROWN MUSHROOM STEW	91
WAX BEANS IN WINE SAUCE	93
LEBANESE MUSHROOM STEW WITH ZA'ATAR	96
SKINNY CUCUMBER NOODLES WITH SAUCE	98
BALKAN-STYLE STIR-FRY	100
ITALIAN ZOODLES WITH ROMANO CHEESE	103

Lime Brussels Sprouts

Prep Time: 10 min | **Cook Time:** 20 min | **Serve:** 4

- 2 pounds Brussels sprouts, trimmed and halved
- 1 tablespoon olive oil
- 2 tablespoons lime juice
- 1 teaspoon lime zest, grated
- 1 teaspoon ground paprika

1. Mix Brussel sprouts with olive oil, lime juice, lime zest, and ground paprika.
2. Put the vegetables in the lined with the baking paper tray and bake for 20 minutes at 365F.

Nutrition: 130 calories, 7.8g protein, 21g carbohydrates, 4.3g fat, 8.8g fiber, 0mg cholesterol, 57mg sodium, 895mg potassium.

Cabbage Bowl

Prep Time: 10 min | **Cook Time:** 20 min | **Serve:** 4

- 4 cups white cabbage
- 1 cup tomatoes, diced
- 2 tablespoons olive oil
- 2 cups of water
- 1 teaspoon dried parsley

1. Mix white cabbage with tomatoes in the saucepan.

2. Add water, dried parsley, and olive oil.

3. Close the lid and simmer the meal on medium heat for 20 minutes.

Nutrition: 86 calories, 1.3g protein, 5.8g carbohydrates, 7.2g fat, 2.3g fiber, 0mg cholesterol, 19mg sodium, 229mg potassium.

Parmesan Asparagus

Prep Time: 10 min | **Cook Time:** 15 min | **Serve:** 4

- 3 oz Parmesan, grated
- 2 tablespoons olive oil
- 1 bunch asparagus, trimmed and halved

1. Line the baking tray with baking paper.

2. Put the asparagus in the tray in one layer and sprinkle it with Parmesan and olive oil.

3. Bake the asparagus at 385F for 15 minutes.

Nutrition: 142 calories, 8.3g protein, 3.4g carbohydrates, 11.6g fat, 1.4g fiber, 15mg cholesterol, 199mg sodium, 135mg potassium.

Coconut Quinoa

Prep Time: 10 min | **Cook Time:** 25 min | **Serve:** 4

- 1 cup quinoa
- 2 cups of water
- 1 cup of coconut milk
- 1 teaspoon ground turmeric

1. Mix water with quinoa and coconut milk.

2. Add ground turmeric and close cook the meal on low heat for 25 minutes.

Nutrition: 296 calories, 7.4g protein, 31g carbohydrates, 16.9g fat, 4.4g fiber, 0mg cholesterol, 15mg sodium, 412mg potassium.

Rosemary Black Beans

Prep Time: 10 min | **Cook Time:** 0 min | **Serve:** 4

- 1 tablespoon avocado oil
- 2 cups canned black beans, drained and rinsed
- 1 tablespoon dried rosemary
- 1 tablespoon lemon juice
- 1 onion, sliced

1. Mix black beans with dried rosemary and lemon juice.
2. Add onion and avocado oil. Shake the meal well.

Nutrition: 350 calories, 21.4g protein, 63.9g carbohydrates, 2g fat, 15.9g fiber, 0mg cholesterol, 7mg sodium, 1502mg potassium.

Oregano Green Beans

Prep Time: 10 min | **Cook Time:** 15 min | **Serve:** 4

- 1 pound green beans, trimmed and halved
- 1 cup of water
- 1 tablespoon dried oregano
- 1 teaspoon chili powder
- 1 tablespoon almond butter

1. Bring the water to boil.
2. Add green beans and boil them for 10 minutes.
3. Then transfer the green beans in the bowl and add dried oregano, chili powder, and almond butter.
4. Stir the meal well.

Nutrition: 65 calories, 3.1g protein, 9.9g carbohydrates, 2.6g fat, 5g fiber, 0mg cholesterol, 16mg sodium, 299mg potassium.

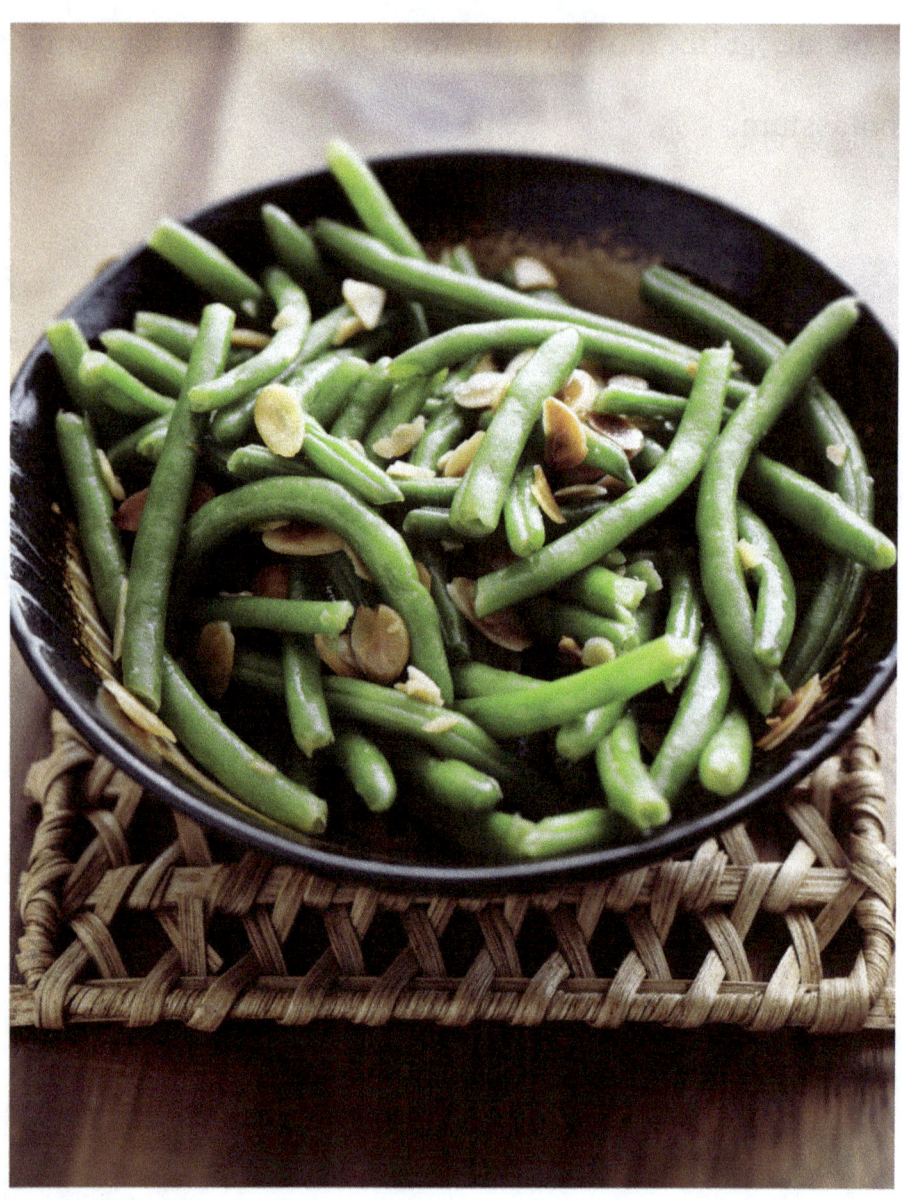

Yam Mash

Prep Time: 10 min | **Cook Time:** 25 min | **Serve:** 4

- 1-pound yams, peeled
- ¼ cup coconut cream
- 1 tablespoon dried dill
-

1. Bake the yams at 365F for 25 minutes.

2. Then mash the yams and mix them with coconut cream and dried dill. Stir the meal well.

Nutrition: 168 calories, 2.2g protein, 32.4g carbohydrates, 3.8g fat, 4.9g fiber, 0mg cholesterol, 13mg sodium, 825mg potassium.

Soft Peas

Prep Time: 10 min | **Cook Time:** 20 min | **Serve:** 4

- 1 cup coconut cream
- 2 cups green peas
- ¼ cup fresh cilantro, chopped

1. Pour coconut cream in the saucepan.

2. Add green peas and cilantro.

3. Close the lid and cook the meal on medium heat for 20 minutes.

Nutrition: 197 calories, 5.3g protein, 13.8g carbohydrates, 14.6g fat, 5.1g fiber, 0mg cholesterol, 13mg sodium, 340mg potassium.

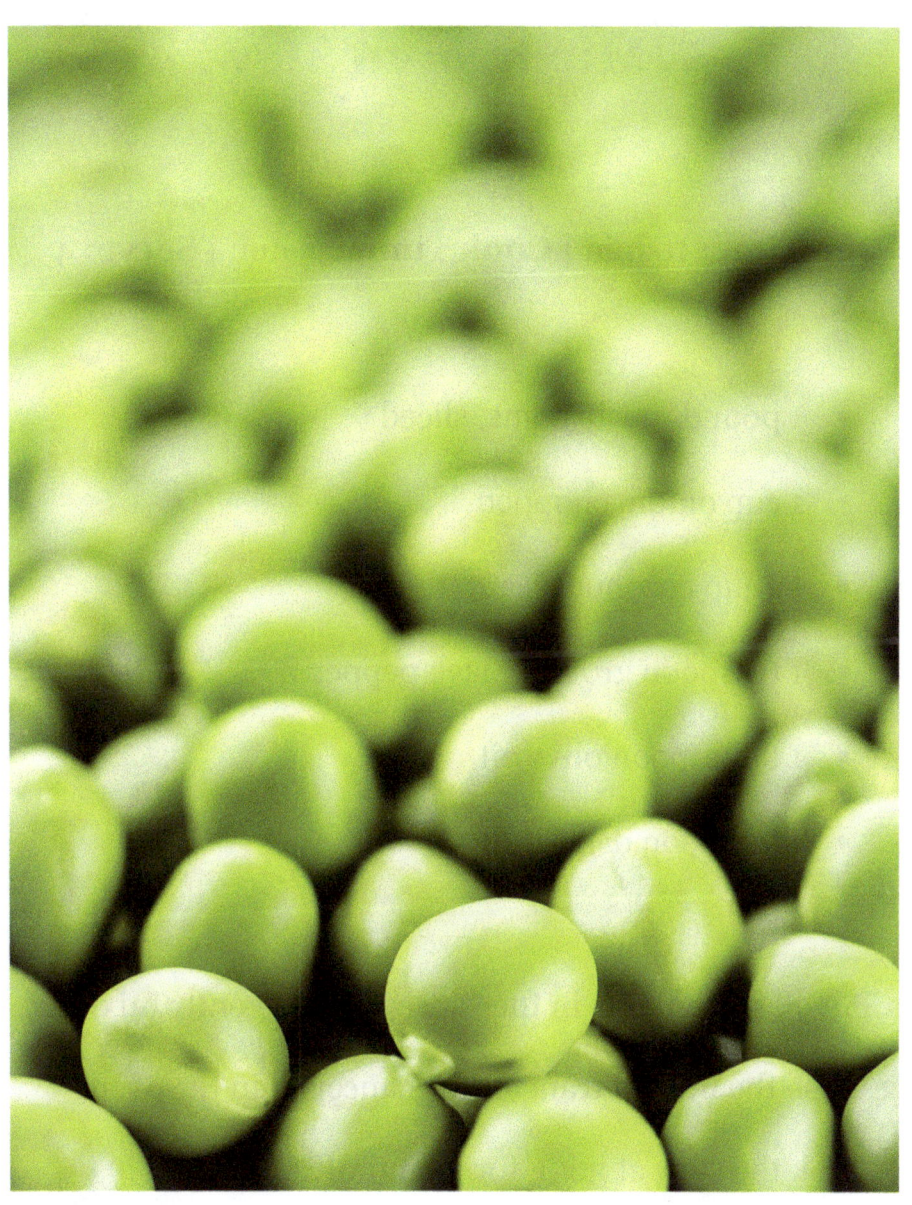

Mushroom Stew

Prep Time: 10 min | **Cook Time:** 35 min | **Serve:** 4

- 1 pound mushrooms, sliced
- 1 cup onion, chopped
- ½ cup coconut cream
- 1 teaspoon ground black pepper
- 1 tablespoon olive oil
- 1 teaspoon dried dill

1. Put all ingredients in the saucepan and gently mix.
2. Close the lid and transfer the saucepan in the oven.
3. Cook the stew at 365F for 35 minutes.

Nutrition: 137 calories, 4.7g protein, 8.6g carbohydrates, 1g fat, 2.6g fiber, 0mg cholesterol, 13mg sodium, 496mg potassium.

Cheesy Broccoli

Prep Time: 10 min | **Cook Time:** 25 min | **Serve:** 4

- 1 pound broccoli florets
- 3 oz Romano cheese, grated
- 1 tablespoon olive oil
- ½ teaspoon ground paprika

1. Line the baking tray with baking paper.

2. Put the broccoli florets inside and sprinkle them with olive oil and ground paprika.

3. Cook the broccoli for 20 minutes at 365F.

4. Then top the vegetables with Romano cheese and bake for 5 minutes more.

Nutrition: 152 calories, 10g protein, 8.4g carbohydrates, 9.6g fat, 3.1g fiber, 22mg cholesterol, 293mg sodium, 383mg potassium.

Glazed Broccoli

Prep Time: 10 min | **Cook Time:** 20 min | **Serve:** 4

- 1 tablespoon avocado oil
- 1 pound broccoli florets
- 1 tablespoon raw honey
- 1 tablespoon rosemary, chopped
- 1 teaspoon chili powder

1. Preheat the skillet well.

2. Add broccoli florets and sprinkle them with avocado oil.

3. Add chili powder and rosemary.

4. Roast the broccoli for 7 minutes per side.

5. Then add honey, carefully mix the vegetables and cook them for 3 minutes more.

Nutrition: 64 calories, 3.4g protein, 13g carbohydrates, 1.1g fat, 3.7g fiber, 0mg cholesterol, 45mg sodium, 393mg potassium.

Cinnamon Asparagus

Prep Time: 10 min | **Cook Time:** 20 min | **Serve:** 4

- 1 pound asparagus, trimmed and halved
- 1 teaspoon ground cinnamon
- 1 tablespoon olive oil
- 1 teaspoon chili flakes
- 1 teaspoon lemon zest, grated

1. Mix asparagus with all remaining ingredients and put in the baking tray.
2. Flatten the asparagus in one layer and bake at 375F for 20 minutes.

Nutrition: 55 calories, 2.5g protein, 5g carbohydrates, 3.7g fat, 2.7g fiber, 0mg cholesterol, 2mg sodium, 234mg potassium.

Spicy Cucumbers

Prep Time: 15 min | **Cook Time:** 0 min | **Serve:** 4

- 3 cups cucumbers, chopped
- 3 tablespoons lemon juice
- 1 tablespoon olive oil
- 1 teaspoon ground coriander
- 1 teaspoon chili powder
- 1 teaspoon dried parsley

1. Put the cucumbers in the big glass jar.

2. Add all remaining ingredients and carefully mix the mixture.

3. Leave it for at least 10 minutes to marinate.

Nutrition: 47 calories, 0.7g protein, 3.5g carbohydrates, 3.8g fat, 0.7g fiber, 0mg cholesterol, 11mg sodium, 143mg potassium.

Spring Salad

Prep Time: 10 min | **Cook Time:** 0 min | **Serve:** 4

- 1 pound cherry tomatoes, halved
- 2 sweet peppers, chopped
- 1 cucumber, chopped
- 2 tablespoons olive oil
- 2 garlic cloves, diced

1. Mix cherry tomatoes with sweet peppers, cucumber, and garlic cloves.
2. Add olive oil and mix the salad well.

Nutrition: 113 calories, 2.2g protein, 12.1g carbohydrates, 7.5g fat, 2.6g fiber, 0mg cholesterol, 9mg sodium, 497mg potassium.

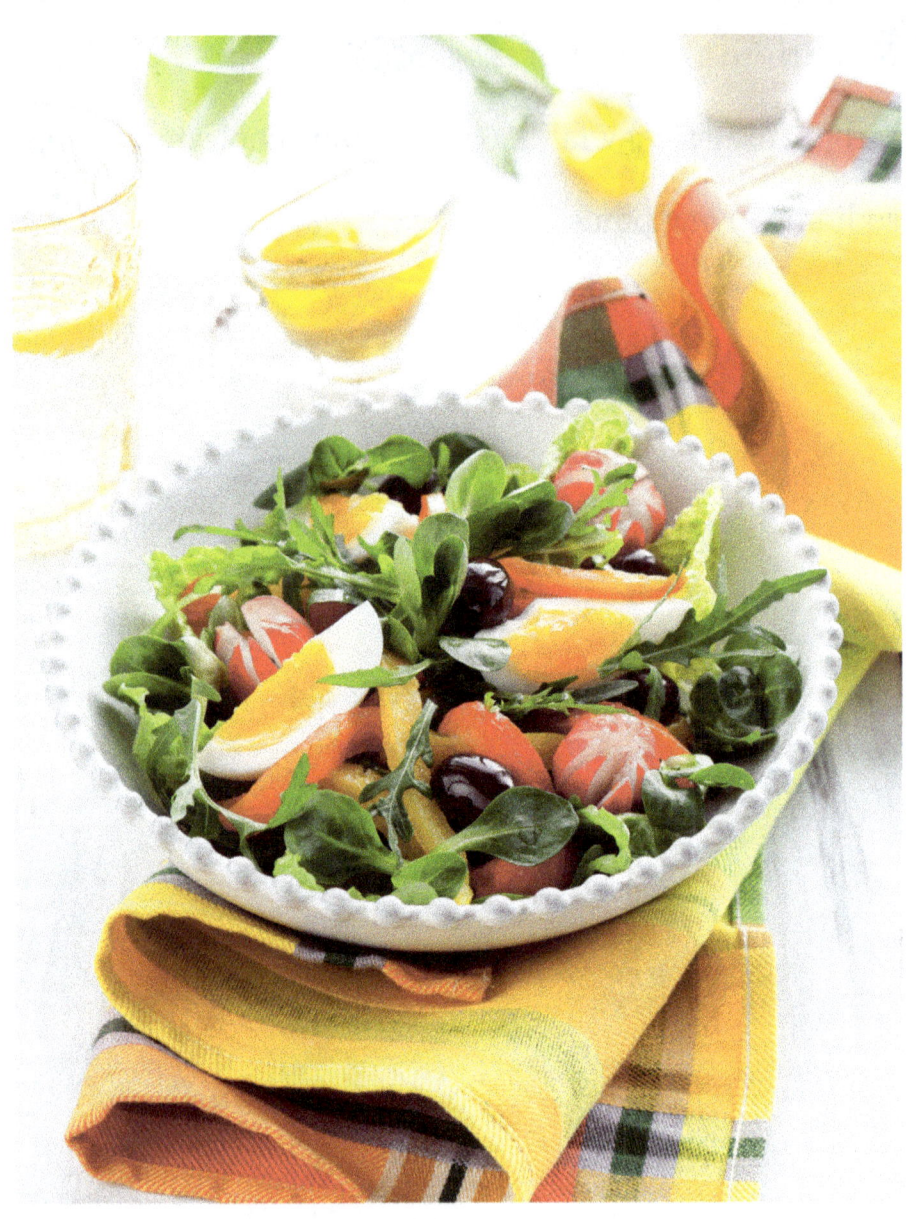

Tender Quinoa

Prep Time: 10 min | **Cook Time:** 30 min | **Serve:** 4

- 1 tablespoon olive oil
- 1 cup quinoa
- 2 cups of water
- 3 tablespoons almond butter

1. Mix quinoa with olive oil and put it in the saucepan.

2. Add water and boil it for 25 minutes on low heat.

3. Then add almond butter and cook the quinoa for 5 minutes more.

Nutrition: 260 calories, 8.6g protein, 29.5g carbohydrates, 12.8g fat, 4.2g fiber, 0mg cholesterol, 7mg sodium, 330mg potassium.

Chickpeas Bowl

Prep Time: 5 min | **Cook Time:** 0 min | **Serve:** 4

- 2 cups canned chickpeas, drained and rinsed
- 1 tomato, chopped
- 1 cup fresh cilantro, chopped
- 1 tablespoon olive oil
- 2 garlic cloves, sliced
- 2 tablespoons lemon juice

1.Mix chickpeas with tomatoes, cilantro, olive oil, garlic, and lemon juice.

2.Stir the mixture well and divide into serving bowls.

Nutrition: 402 calories, 19.7g protein, 62.1g carbohydrates, 9.7g fat, 17.8g fiber, 0mg cholesterol, 28mg sodium, 948mg potassium.

Beans Mash

Prep Time: 10 min | **Cook Time:** 0 min | **Serve:** 4

- 16 oz white beans, boiled
- 1 tablespoon almond butter
- ¼ cup coconut cream
- ½ teaspoon ground clove

1. Put the white beans in the blender.

2. Add almond butter, coconut cream, and ground clove.

3. Blend the mixture until smooth and transfer into the serving bowls.

Nutrition: 437 calories, 27.7g protein, 70.1g carbohydrates, 6.8g fat, 18.1g fiber, mg cholesterol, 21mg sodium, 2108mg potassium.

Spiralized Carrot

Prep Time: 5 min | **Cook Time:** 5 min | **Serve:** 4

- 7 carrots, spiralized
- 2 tablespoons lime juice
- 1 tablespoon olive oil
- 1 teaspoon ground black pepper

1. Preheat the olive oil in the skillet well.
2. Add carrot and ground black pepper.
3. Roast the carrot for 2-3 minutes.
4. Add lime juice, stir the carrot, and cook it for 2 minutes more.

Nutrition: 77 calories, 1g protein, 11.4g carbohydrates, 3.5g fat, 2.8g fiber, 0mg cholesterol, 75mg sodium, 354mg potassium.

Classic Barley

Prep Time: 5 min | **Cook Time:** 30 min | **Serve:** 4

- 2 cups barley
- 4 cups of water
- 1 tablespoon olive oil

1. Mix water with barley and olive oil.
2. Cook the barley with the closed lid for 30 minutes on low heat.

Nutrition: 356 calories, 11.5g protein, 67.6g carbohydrates, 5.6g fat, 15.9g fiber, 0mg cholesterol, 18mg sodium, 418mg potassium.

Baked Mango

Prep Time: 5 min | **Cook Time:** 20 min | **Serve:** 4

- 2 mangos, peeled and chopped
- 1 tablespoon Italian seasonings
- 1 tablespoon olive oil

1. Mix mango with Italian seasonings and olive oil.

2. Put the mango in the tray and bake it for 20 minutes at 355F.

Nutrition: 131 calories, 1.4g protein, 25.2g carbohydrates, 4.1g fat, 2.7g fiber, 0mg cholesterol, 2mg sodium, 282mg potassium.

Easy Cabbage Slaw

Prep Time: 10 min | **Cook Time:** 0 min | **Serve:** 4

- 2 cups green cabbage, shredded
- 1 carrot, grate
- 3 tablespoons raisins, chopped
- 2 tablespoons coconut cream
- 1 tablespoon lemon juice
- 1 tablespoon olive oil

1. Mix green cabbage with carrot, raisins, coconut cream, and lemon juice.
2. Then add olive oil and carefully mix the slaw.

Nutrition: 83 calories, 1g protein, 9.4g carbohydrates, 5.4g fat, 1.7g fiber, 0mg cholesterol, 19mg sodium, 184mg potassium.

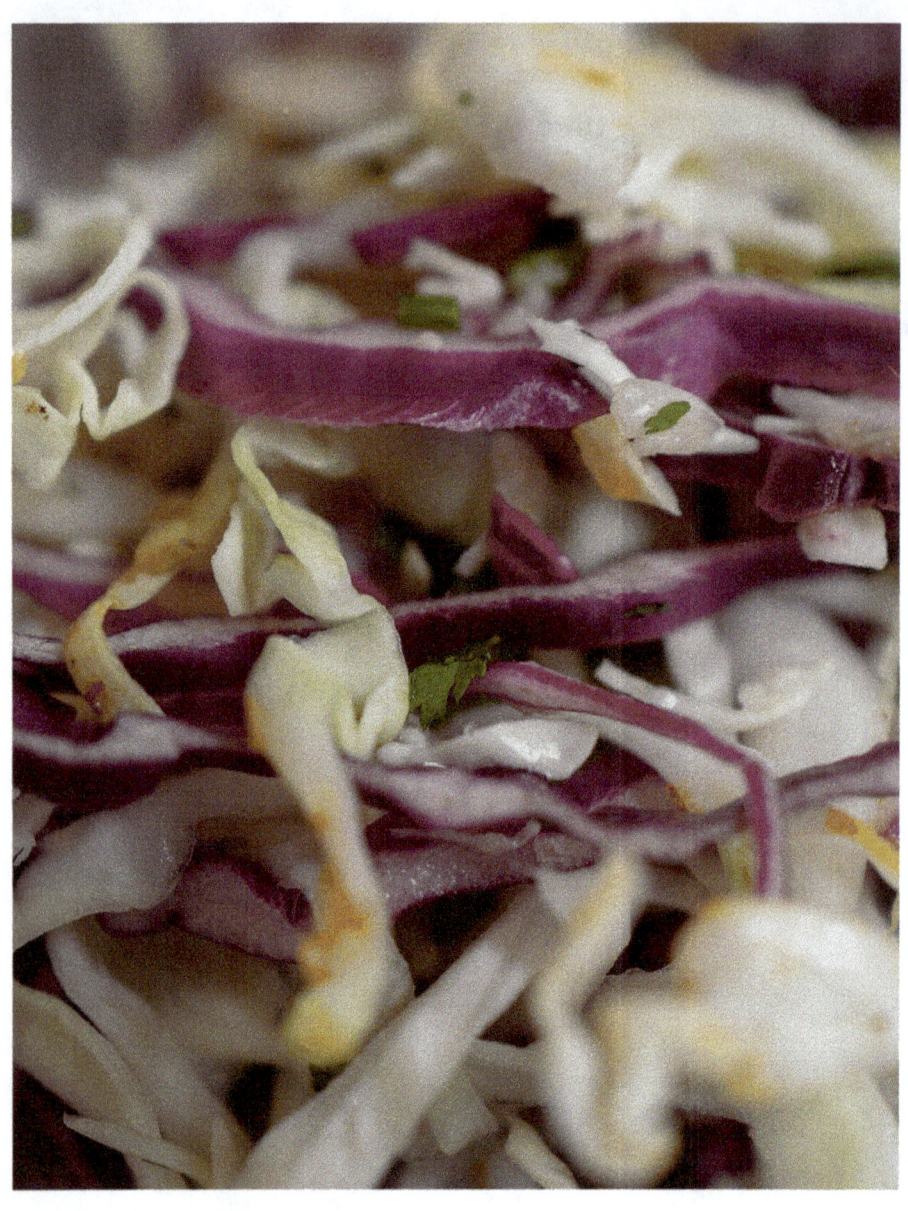

Apple Salad

Prep Time: 5 min | **Cook Time:** 0 min | **Serve:** 4

- 5 apples, chopped
- ½ cup fresh dill, chopped
- 1 tablespoon olive oil
- 1 tomato, chopped

1.Mix apples with dill and tomato.

2.Add olive oil and stir the salad one more time.

Nutrition: 193 calories, 2.1g protein, 42.5g carbohydrates, 4.3g fat, 7.8g fiber, 0mg cholesterol, 16mg sodium, 533mg potassium.

Avocado Mash

Prep Time: 10 min | **Cook Time:** 0 min | **Serve:** 4

- 1 tablespoon fresh cilantro, chopped
- 2 avocados, peeled, pitted and sliced
- 1 tablespoon minced garlic
- 2 tablespoons lemon juice
- 1 tablespoon olive oil

1. Blend the avocado until smooth and transfer it in the bowl.
2. Add cilantro, minced garlic, lemon juice, and olive oil.
3. Stir the meal well.

Nutrition: 240 calories, 2.1g protein, 9.5g carbohydrates, 23.2g fat, 6.8g fiber, 0mg cholesterol, 8mg sodium, 507mg potassium.

Bake Endives

Prep Time: 10 min | **Cook Time:** 20 min | **Serve:** 4

- 1-pound endives, roughly chopped
- 1 tablespoon olive oil
- 1 tablespoon garlic powder

1. Put the endives in the baking tray.

2. Sprinkle the vegetables with olive oil and garlic powder.

3. Bake the endives at 365F for 20 minutes.

Nutrition: 56 calories, 1.8g protein, 5.3g carbohydrates, 3.8g fat, 3.7g fiber, 0mg cholesterol, 26mg sodium, 379mg potassium.

Arugula Bowl

Prep Time: 5 min | **Cook Time:** 0 min | **Serve:** 4

- 2 cups baby arugula
- Juice of 1 lime
- 1 cup tomatoes, chopped
- 3 oz Romano cheese, crumbled
- 1 tablespoon olive oil

1. Put all ingredients in the bowl.
2. Shake the meal before serving.

Nutrition: 128 calories, 7.7g protein, 4.6g carbohydrates, 9.4g fat, 1.2g fiber, 22mg cholesterol, 260mg sodium, 181mg potassium.

Potato Mash

Prep Time: 15 min | **Cook Time:** 20 min | **Serve:** 32

- 10 large baking potatoes, peeled and cubed
- 3 tablespoons organic olive oil, divided
- 1 onion, chopped
- 1 tablespoon ground turmeric
- ½ teaspoon ground cumin
- Salt and freshly ground black pepper, to taste

1. In a large pan of water, add potatoes and produce with a boil on medium-high heat.
2. Cook approximately twenty or so minutes.
3. Drain well and transfer in to a large bowl.
4. With a potato masher, mash the potatoes.

5. Meanwhile in a very skillet, heat 1 tablespoon of oil on medium-high heat.

6. Add onion and sauté for about 6 minutes.

7. Add onion mixture in the bowl with mashed potatoes.

8. Add turmeric, cumin, salt and black pepper and mash till well combined.

9. Stir in remaining oil and serve.

Nutrition: Calories: 103, Fat: 1.4g, Carbohydrates: 21.3g, Fiber: 2g, Protein: 1.8g

Creamy Sweet Potato Mash

Prep Time: 15 min | **Cook Time:** 21 min | **Serve:** 4

- 1 tbsp. extra virgin olive oil
- 2 large sweet potatoes, peeled and chopped
- 2 teaspoons ground turmeric
- 1 garlic herb, minced
- 2 cups vegetable broth
- 2 tablespoons unsweetened coconut milk Salt and freshly ground black pepper, to taste Chopped pistachios, for garnishing

1. In a big skillet, heat oil on medium-high heat. Add sweet potato and stir fry for bout 2-3 minutes.

2. Add turmeric and stir fry for approximately 1 minute.

3. Add garlic and stir fry approximately 2 minutes.

4. Add broth and provide to a boil.

5. Reduce the heat to low and cook for approximately 10-15 minutes or till

6. every one of the liquids is absorbed.

7. Transfer the sweet potato mixture in to a bowl.

8. Add coconut milk, salt and black pepper and mash it completely.

9. Garnish with pistachio and serve.

Nutrition: Calories: 110, Fat: 5g, Carbohydrates: 16g, Protein: 1g

Gingered Cauliflower Rice

Prep Time: 15 min | **Cook Time:** 10 min | **Serve:** 3-4

- 3 tablespoons coconut oil
- 4 (1/8-inch thickfresh ginger slices
- 1 small head cauliflower, trimmed and processed into rice consistency
- 3 garlic cloves, crushed
- 1 tablespoon chives, chopped
- 1 tablespoon coconut vinegar
- Salt, to taste

1. In a skillet, melt coconut oil on medium-high heat.
2. Add ginger and sauté for about 2-3 minutes.
3. Discard the ginger slices and stir in cauliflower and garlic.

4.Cook, stirring occasionally approximately 7-8 minutes.

5.Stir in remaining ingredients and take off from heat.

Nutrition: Calories: 67, Fat: 3.5g, Carbohydrates: 4.5g, Fiber: 2g, Protein: 7g

Spicy Cauliflower Rice

Prep Time: 15 min | **Cook Time:** 10 min | **Serve:** 4

- 3 tablespoons coconut oil
- 1 small white onion, chopped
- 3 garlic cloves, minced
- 1 large head cauliflower, trimmed and processed into rice consistency
- ½ teaspoon ground cumin
- ½ teaspoon paprika
- Salt and freshly ground black pepper, to taste 1large tomato, chopped
- ¼ cup tomato paste
- ¼ cup fresh cilantro, chopped Chopped fresh cilantro, for garnishing 2 limes, quarters

1. In a sizable skillet, melt coconut oil on medium-high heat.

2. Add onion and sauté for approximately 2 minutes.

3. Add garlic and sauté approximately 1 minute.

4. Stir in cauliflower rice.

5. Add cumin, paprika, salt and black pepper and cook, stirring occasionally approximately 2-3 minutes.

6. Stir in tomato, tomato paste and cilantro and cook approximately 2-3 minutes.

7. Garnish with cilantro and serve alongside lime.

Nutrition: Calories: 246, Fat: 11g, Carbohydrates: 26g, Fiber: 4g, Protein: 21g

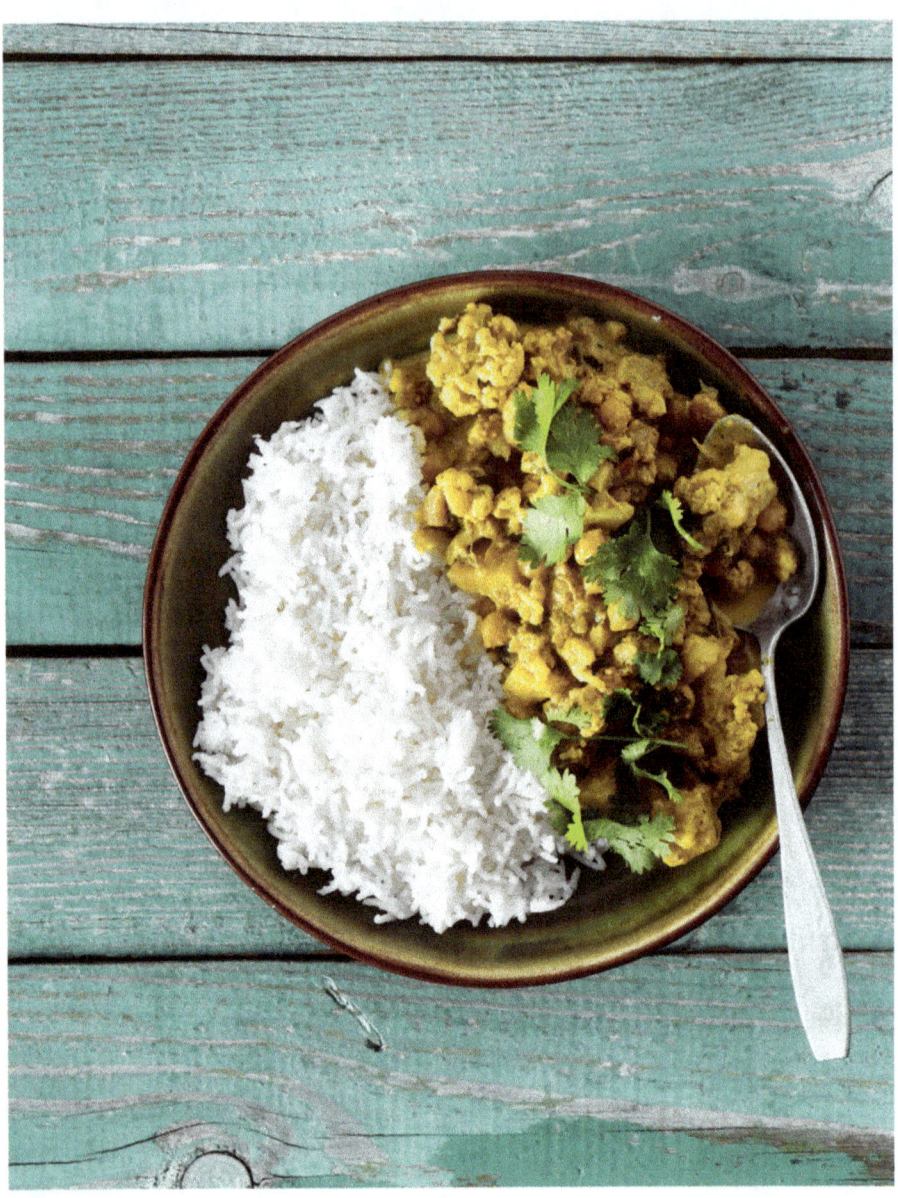

Simple Brown Rice

Prep Time: 10 min | **Cook Time:** 50 min | **Serve:** 4

- 1 cup brown rice
- 2 cups chicken broth
- 1 tablespoon ground turmeric
- 1 tbsp. extra virgin olive oil

1. In a pan, add rice, broth and turmeric and provide with a boil.
2. Reduce the warmth to low.
3. Simmer, covered for about 50 minutes.
4. Add the organic olive oil and fluff using a fork.
5. Keep aside, covered approximately 10 minutes before.

Nutrition: Calories: 320, Fat: 6g, Carbohydrates: 285g, Fiber: 4g, Protein: 21g

Spicy Quinoa

Prep Time: 10 min | **Cook Time:** 25 min | **Serve:** 4

- 2 tablespoons extra-virgin essential olive oil
- 1 teaspoon curry powder
- 1 teaspoon ground turmeric
- 12 teaspoon ground cumin
- 1 cup quinoa, rinsed and drained
- 2 cups chicken broth
- ¾ cup almonds, toasted ½ cup raisins
- ¾ cup fresh parsley, chopped

1. In a medium pan, heat oil on medium-low heat.

2. Add curry powder, turmeric and cumin and sauté for approximately 1-2 minutes.

3. Add quinoa and sauté approximately 2-3 minutes.

4. Add broth and stir to blend.

5. Cover reducing the warmth to low.

6. Simmer for around twenty minutes.

7. Remove from heat while aside, covered approximately 5 minutes.

8. Just before, add almonds and raisins and toss to coat.

10 Drizzle with lemon juice and serve.

Nutrition: Calories: 237, Fat: 3g, Carbohydrates: 17g, Fiber: 6g, Protein: 31g

Quinoa with Apricots

Prep Time: 15 min | **Cook Time:** 12 min | **Serve:** 4

- 2 cups water
- 1 cup quinoa
- ½ teaspoon fresh ginger, grated finely
- ½ cup dried apricots, chopped roughly
- Salt and freshly ground black pepper, to taste

1. In a pan, add water on high heat and bring to your boil.

2. Add quinoa and reduce the heat to medium.

3. Cover and reduce the heat to low.

4. Simmer for about 12 minutes.

5. Remove from heat and immediately, stir in ginger and apricots. Keep aside, covered for approximately fifteen minutes before.

Nutrition: Calories: 267, Fat: 3.5g, Carbohydrates: 4g, Fiber: 5g, Protein: 17g

Easy Zucchini Slaw

Prep Time: 10 min | **Serve:** 3

- 2 tablespoons extra-virgin olive oil
- 1 zucchini, shredded
- 1 teaspoon Dijon mustard
- 1 yellow bell pepper, sliced
- 1 red onion, thinly sliced

1.Combine all ingredients in a salad bowl. Season with the salt and black pepper to taste.

2.Let it sit in your refrigerator for about 1 hour before.

Nutrition: 96 Calories; 9.4g Fat; 2.8g Carbs; 0.7g Protein; 0.4g Fiber Ingredients

Broc n' Cheese

Prep Time: 25 min | **Serve:** 5

- 1 ½ pounds broccoli florets
- 3 tablespoons olive oil
- 1/2 cup cream of mushrooms soup
- 1 teaspoon garlic, minced
- 6 ounces Swiss cheese, shredded

1. Start by preheating your oven to 380 degrees F. Brush the sides and bottom of a baking dish with 1 tablespoon olive oil.

2. In a small nonstick skillet, heat 1 tablespoon of the olive oil over a moderate heat. Sauté the garlic for 30 seconds or until just beginning to brown.

3.In a soup pot, parboil the broccoli until crisp-tender; place the rinsed broccoli in the prepared baking dish. Place the sautéed garlic on top. Drizzle the remaining tablespoon of olive oil over everything.

4.Season with the salt and black pepper. Pour in the cream of mushroom soup.

5.2Top with the Swiss cheese.

6.Bake for 20 minutes until the cheese is hot and bubbly.

Nutrition: 179 Calories; 10.3g Fat; 7.6g Carbs; 13.5g Protein; 3.6g Fiber

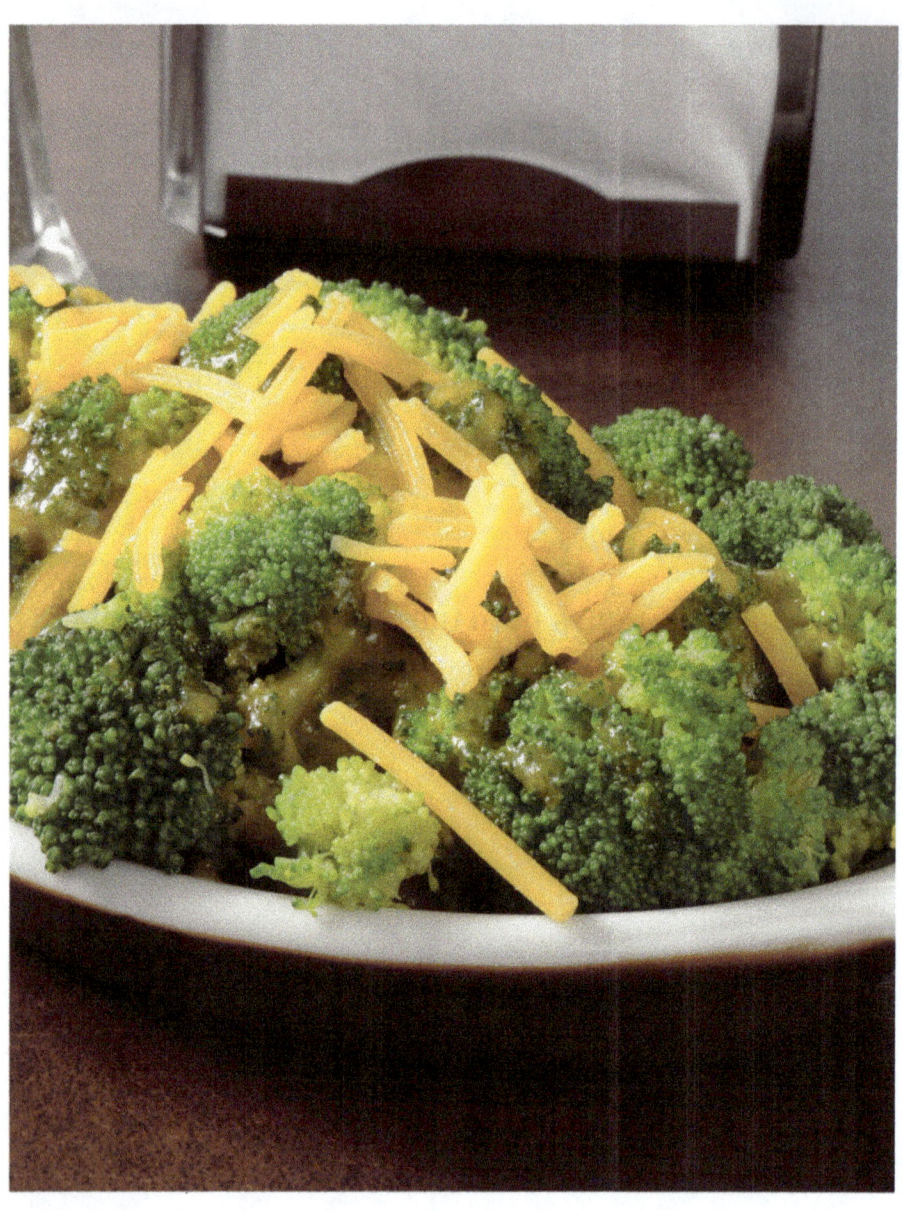

Greek Avgolemono Soup

Prep Time: 25 min | **Serve:** 6

- 1 pound fennel bulbs, sliced
- 1 celery stalk, chopped
- 1 tablespoon freshly squeezed lemon juice
- 2 eggs
- 5 cups chicken stock

1. Heat 2 tablespoons of olive oil in a soup pot over medium-high heat. Sauté the fennel and celery until tender but not browned, approximately 7 minutes.
2. Add in Mediterranean seasoning mix and continue to sauté until they are fragrant.

3. Add in the chicken stock and bring to a rapid boil. Turn the temperature to medium-low; let it simmer for 10 to 13 minutes.

4. Puree your soup using a food processor or an immersion blender.

5. Thoroughly whisk the eggs and lemon juice until well combined; pour 2 cups of the hot soup into the egg mixture, whisking continuously.

Return the mixture to the pot; continue cooking for 2 to 3 minutes more until cooked through. Spoon into individual bowls.

Nutrition: 86 Calories; 6.1g Fat; 6g Carbs; 2.8g Protein; 2.4g Fiber

Italian Zuppa Di Pomodoro

Prep Time: 35 minutes | **Serve:** 4

- 1/2 cup scallions, chopped
- 1 ½ pounds Roma tomatoes, diced
- 2 cups Brodo di Pollo (Italian broth
- 2 tablespoons tomato paste
- 2 cups mustard greens, torn into pieces

1.Heat 2 teaspoon of olive oil in a large pot over medium-high heat. Sauté the scallions for 2 to 3 minutes until tender.

2.Add in Roma tomatoes, Italian broth, and tomato paste and bring to a boil. Reduce the temperature to medium-low and continue to simmer, partially covered, for about 25 minutes.

3.Puree the soup with an immersion blender and return it to the pot. Add in the mustard greens and continue to cook until the greens wilt.

4.Taste, adjust seasonings and serve immediately.

Nutrition: 104 Calories; 7.2g Fat; 6.2g Carbs; 2.6g Protein; 3.1g Fiber

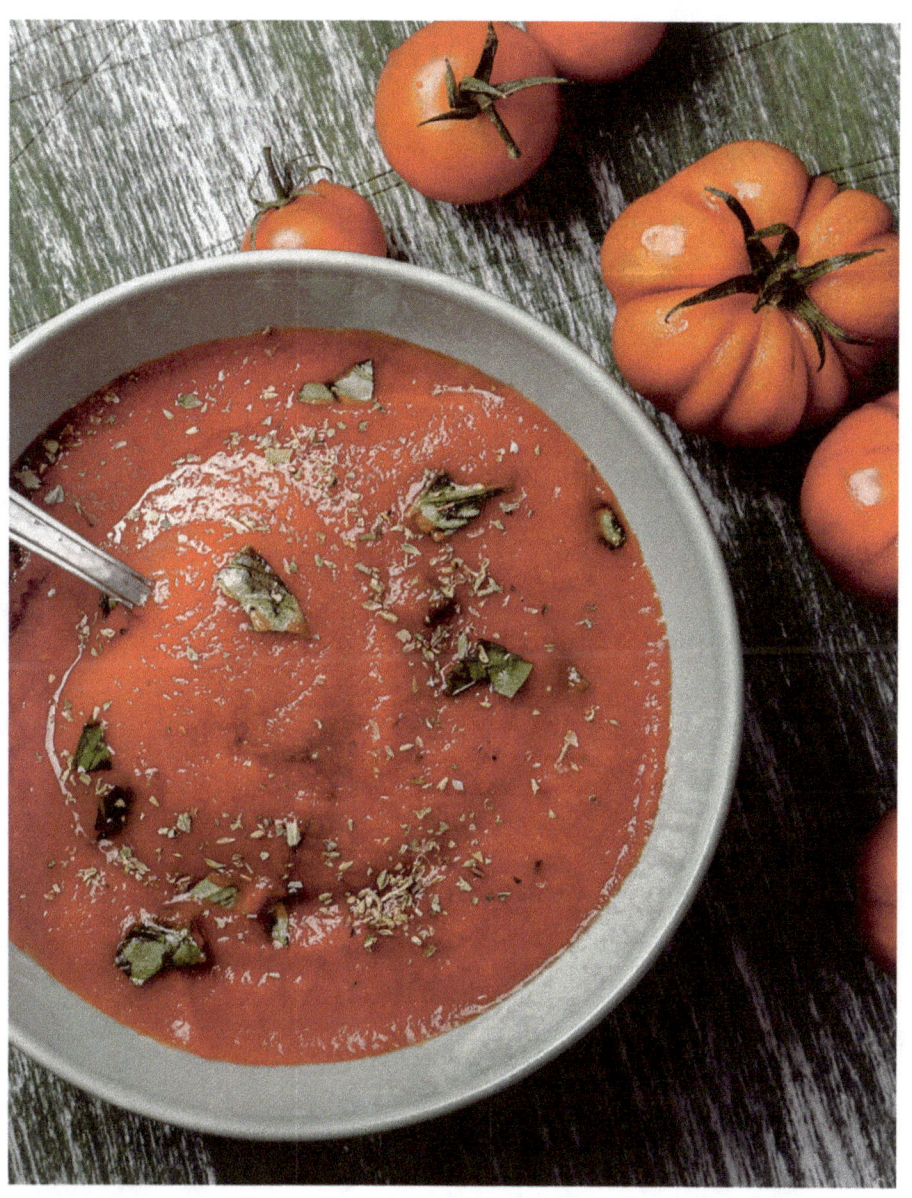

Easy Zucchini Croquets

Prep Time: 40 minutes | **Serve:** 6

- 1 egg
- 1/2 cup almond meal
- 1 pound zucchini, grated and drained
- 1/2 cup goat cheese, crumbled
- 2 tablespoons olive oil

1.Combine the egg, almond milk, zucchini and cheese in a mixing bowl.

2.Refrigerate the mixture for 20 to 30 minutes.

3.Heat the oil in a frying pan over medium-high heat. Scoop the heaped tablespoons of the mixture into the hot oil.

4.Cook for about 4 minutes per side; cook in batches.

Nutrition: 111 Calories; 8.9g Fat; 3.2g Carbs; 5.8g Protein; 1g Fiber

Pork and Cheese Stuffed Peppers

Prep Time: 30 minutes | **Serve:** 2

- 2 sweet Italian peppers, deveined and halved
- 1/2 Spanish onion, finely chopped
- 1 cup marinara sauce
- 1/2 cup cheddar cheese, grated
- 4 ounces pork, ground

1.Heat 1 tablespoon of canola oil in a saucepan over a moderate heat. Then, sauté the onion for 3 to 4 minutes until tender and fragrant.

2.Add in the ground pork; cook for 3 to 4 minutes more. Add in Italian seasoning mix. Spoon the mixture into the pepper halves.

3.Spoon the marinara sauce into a lightly greased baking dish. Arrange the stuffed peppers in the baking dish.

4.Bake in the preheated oven at 395 degrees F for 17 to 20 minutes. Top with cheddar cheese and continue to bake for about 5 minutes or until the top is golden brown. Bon appétit!

Nutrition: 313 Calories; 21.3g Fat; 5.7g Carbs; 20.2g Protein; 1.9g Fiber

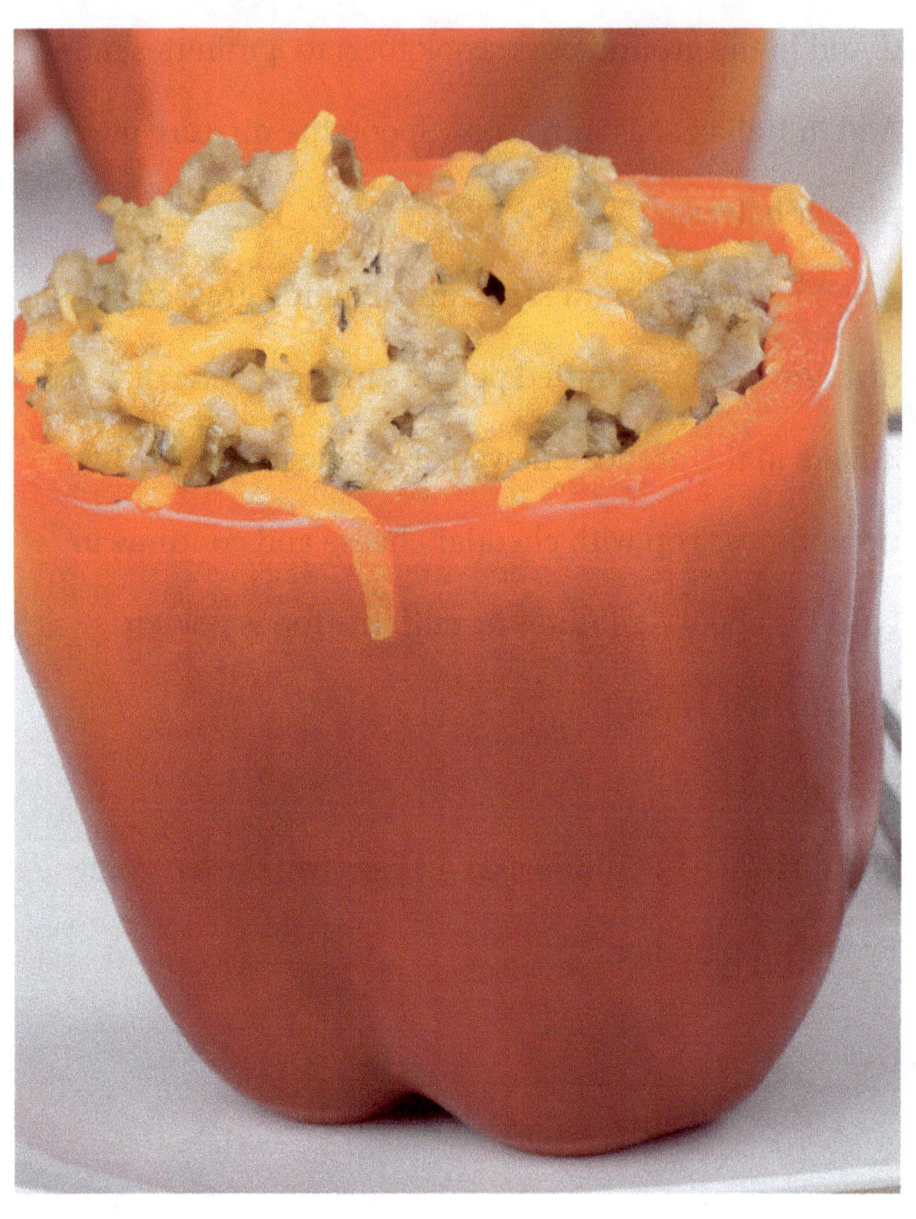

Stewed Cabbage with Goan Chorizo Sausage

Prep Time: 30 minutes | **Serve:** 3

- 6 ounces Goan chorizo sausage, sliced
- 3/4 cup cream of celery soup
- 1-pound white cabbage, outer leaves removed and finely shredded
- 2 cloves garlic, finely chopped
- 1 teaspoon Indian spice blend

1. In a large frying pan, sear the sausage until no longer pink; set aside.

2.Then, sauté the garlic and Indian spice blend until they are aromatic. Add in the cabbage and cream of celery soup.

3.Turn the heat to simmer; continue to simmer, partially covered, for about 20 minutes or until cooked through.

4.Top with the reserved Goan chorizo sausage and serve.

Nutrition: 235 Calories; 17.7g Fat; 6.1g Carbs; 9.8g Protein; 2.4g Fiber

Cauliflower and Ham Casserole

Prep Time: 10 min | **Serve:** 6

- 1 ½ pounds cauliflower, broken into small florets
- 6 ounces ham, diced
- 4 eggs, beaten
- 1/2 cup Greek-Style yogurt
- 1 cup Swiss cheese, preferably freshly grated

1. Parboil the cauliflower in a saucepan for about 10 minutes or until tender.

2. Drain and puree in your food processor.

3.Add in the ham, eggs, and Greek-Style yogurt; stir to combine well.

4.Spoon the mixture into a lightly buttered baking dish. Top with the Swiss cheese and bake in the preheated oven at 385 degrees F for about 20 minutes.

Nutrition: 236 Calories; 13.8g Fat; 7.2g Carbs; 20.3g Protein; 2.3g Fiber

Stuffed Spaghetti Squash

Prep Time: 1 hour | **Serve:** 4

- ½ pound spaghetti squash, halved, scoop out seeds
- 1 garlic clove, minced
- 1 cup cream cheese
- 2 eggs
- 1/2 cup Mozzarella cheese, shredded

1. Drizzle the insides of each squash with 1 teaspoon of olive oil. Bake in the preheated oven at 380 degrees F for 45 minutes.

2. Scrape out the spaghetti squash "noodles" from the skin. Fold in the remaining ingredients; stir to combine well.

3.Spoon the cheese mixture into squash halves. Bake at 360 degrees F for about 9 minutes, until the cheese is hot and bubbly.

Nutrition: 219 Calories; 17.5g Fat; 6.9g Carbs; 9g Protein; 0.9g Fiber

Spicy and Warm Coleslaw

Prep Time: 45 min | **Serve:** 4

- 1 medium-sized leek, chopped
- 1 tablespoon balsamic vinegar
- 1 teaspoon yellow mustard
- ½ pound green cabbage, shredded
- ½ teaspoon Sriracha sauce

1. Drizzle 2 tablespoons of the olive oil over the leek and cabbage; sprinkle with salt and black pepper.
2. Bake in the preheated oven at 410 degrees F for about 40 minutes. Transfer the mixture to a salad bowl.
3. Toss with 1 tablespoon of olive oil, mustard, balsamic vinegar, and Sriracha sauce. Serve warm!

Nutrition: 118 Calories; 10.2g Fat; 6.6g Carbs; 1.1g Protein; 1.9g Fiber

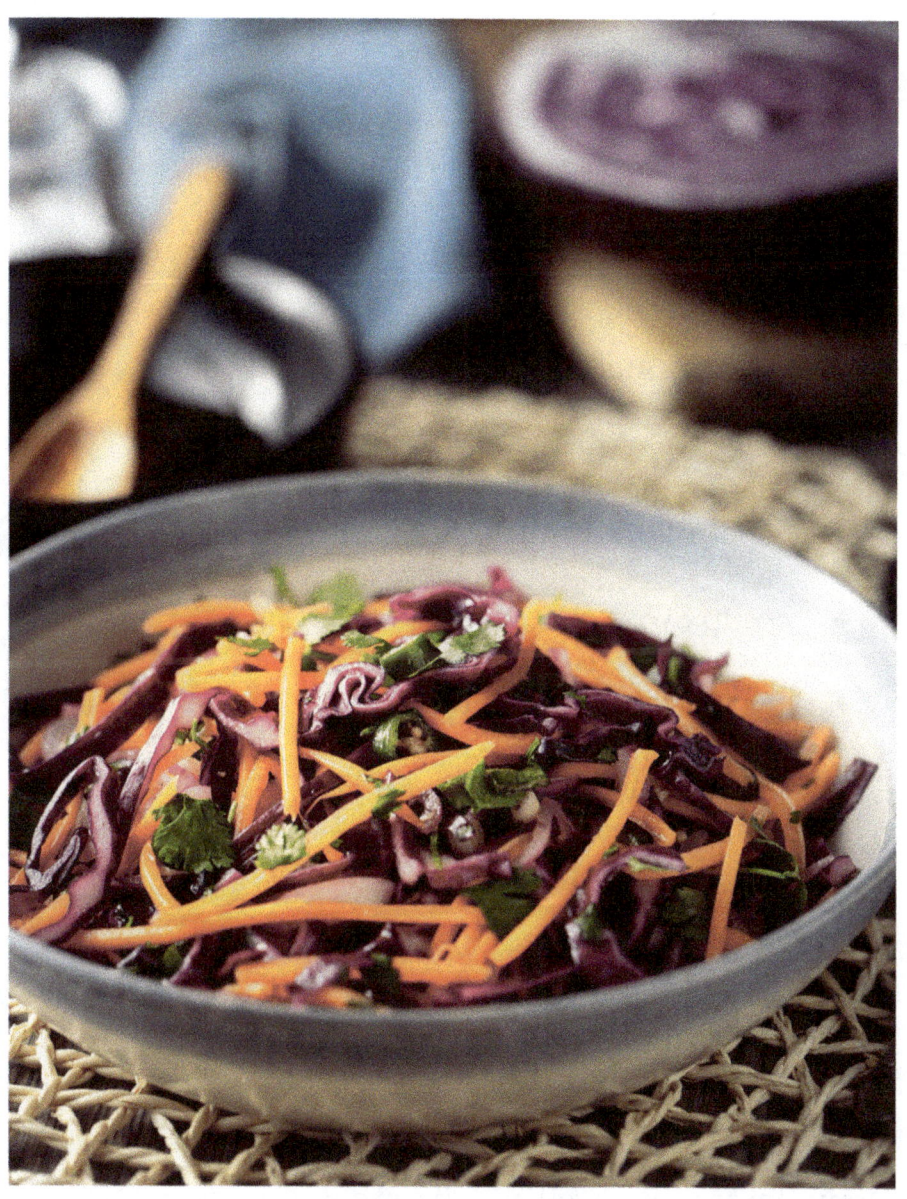

Easy Mediterranean Croquettes

Prep Time: 40minutes | **Serve:** 2

- ½ pound zucchini, grated
- ½ cup Swiss cheese, shredded
- 3 eggs, whisked Mediterranean
- 1/3 cup almond meal
- 2 tablespoons pork rinds

1.Place the grated zucchini in a colander, sprinkle with 1/2 teaspoon of salt, and let it stand for 30 minutes. Drain the zucchini well and discard any excess water.

2.Heat 2 tablespoons of olive oil in a frying pan over medium-high heat. Mix the zucchini with the remaining ingredients until well combined.

3.Shape the mixture into croquettes and cook for 2 to 3 minutes per side. Enjoy!

Nutrition: 463 Calories; 36g Fat; 7.6g Carbs; 27.5g Protein; 2.8g Fiber

Tuscan Asparagus with Cheese

Prep Time: 20 min | **Serve:** 5

- 1 ½ pounds asparagus, trimmed
- 1 tablespoon Sriracha sauce
- 1 tablespoon fresh cilantro, roughly chopped
- 4 tablespoons Pecorino Romano cheese, grated
- 4 tablespoons butter, melted

1. Toss the asparagus with the cheese, melted butter, and Sriracha sauce; season with Italian spice mix, if desired.
2. Arrange your asparagus on a baking sheet and roast in the preheated oven at 410 degrees F for 12 to 15 minutes.
3. Garnish with fresh cilantro and enjoy!

Nutrition: 140 Calories; 11.5g Fat; 5.5g Carbs; 5.6g Protein; 2.9g Fiber

Brown Mushroom Stew

Prep Time: 20 min | **Serve:** 6

- 2 pounds brown mushrooms, sliced
- 1 bell pepper, sliced
- 2 cups chicken broth
- ½ cup leeks, finely diced
- 1 cup herb-infused tomato sauce

1. Heat 4 tablespoons of oil in a soup pot over a moderate flame. Sauté the pepper and leeks for about 4 to 5 minutes.
2. Stir in the mushrooms and continue to sauté for about 2 minutes. Pour in a splash of broth to deglaze the bottom of the pan.
3. After that, add in the tomato sauce and the remaining broth; bring to a boil.

4.Turn the heat to simmer.

5.Continue to cook, partially covered, for about 10 minutes or until the mushrooms are tender and thoroughly cooked.

6.Ladle into soup bowls and serve. Bon appétit!

Nutrition: 123 Calories; 9.2g Fat; 5.8g Carbs; 4.7g Protein; 1.4g Fiber

Wax Beans in Wine Sauce

Prep Time: 15 minutes | **Serve:** 4

- ½ pound wax beans, trimmed
- 2 tablespoons dry white wine
- 1 tablespoon butter
- ½ teaspoon mustard seeds
- ½ cup tomato sauce with garlic and onions

1. Melt the butter in a soup pot over medium-high heat. Then, fry wax beans in hot butter for 2 to 3 minutes.
2. Add in tomato sauce, wine, and mustard seeds; season with salt and black pepper.
3. Turn the temperature to medium-low and continue to simmer for about 8 longer or until wax beans are tender

and the sauce has thickened slightly. Bon appétit!

Nutrition: 56 Calories; 3.5g Fat; 6g Carbs; 1.5g Protein; 2.2g Fiber

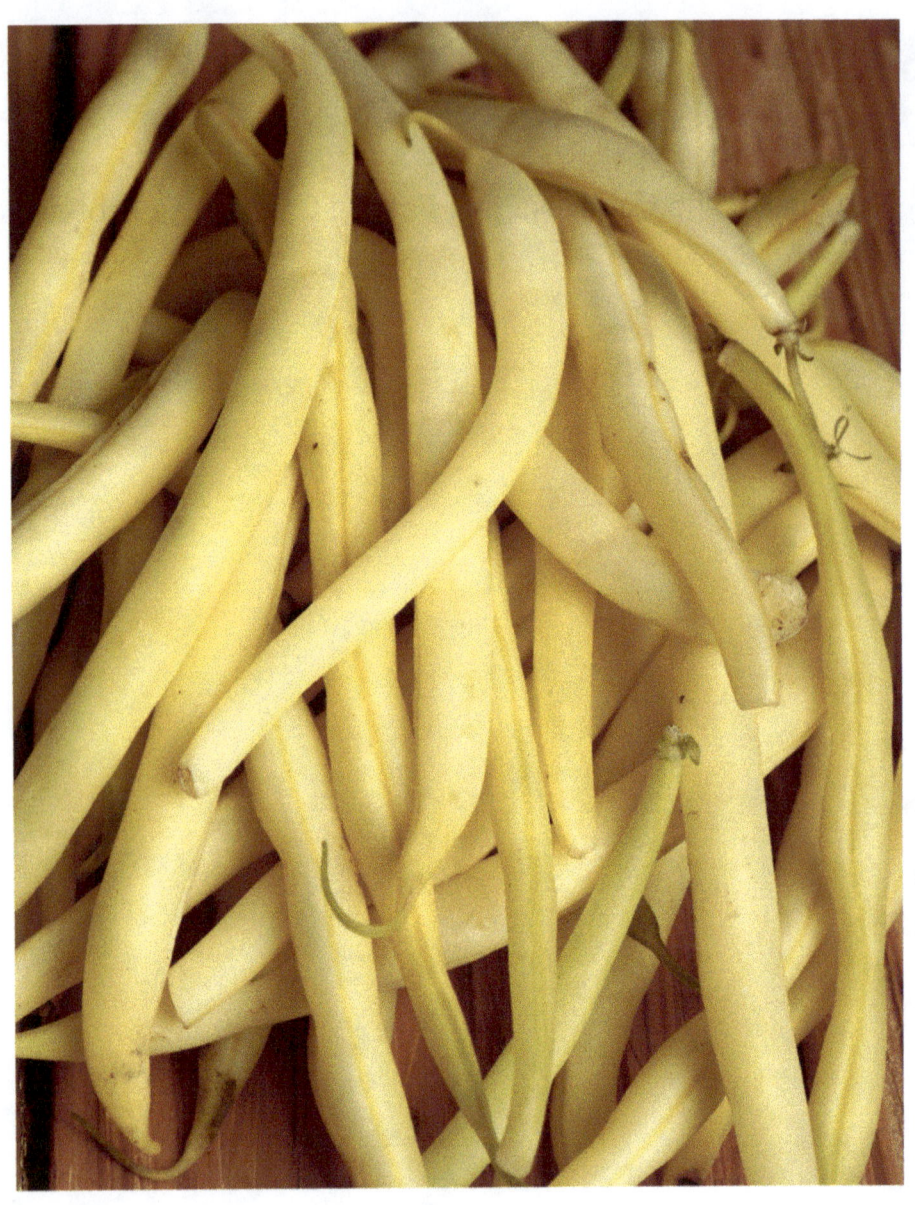

Lebanese Mushroom Stew with Za'atar

Prep Time: 1 hour 50 minutes | **Serve:** 4

- 8 ounces Chanterelle mushroom, sliced
- 1 cup tomato sauce with onion and garlic
- 4 tablespoons olive oil
- 2 bell peppers, chopped
- ½ teaspoon Za'atar spice

1. Heat olive oil in a heavy-bottomed pot over medium-high heat. Once hot, sauté the peppers until tender or about 3 minutes.

2. Stir in the mushrooms and continue to sauté until they have softened

3. Add in Za'atar spice and tomato sauce; bring to a rapid boil. Immediately, turn the heat to medium-low.

4. Continue to simmer for about 35 minutes until cooked through. Bon appétit!

Nutrition: 155 Calories; 13.9g Fat; 6g Carbs; 1.4g Protein; 2.9g Fiber

Skinny Cucumber Noodles with Sauce

Prep Time: 35 minutes | **Serve:** 2

- 1 cucumber, spiralized
- ½ teaspoon sea salt
- 1 tablespoon olive oil
- 1 tablespoon fresh lime juice
- 1 California avocado, pitted, peeled and mashed

1. Sprinkle your cucumber with salt; let it stand for 30 minutes; after that, discard the excess water and pat the cucumber dry with kitchen towels.

2. In the meantime, combine olive oil, lime juice, and avocado. Season with salt and black pepper.

3.Toss the cucumber noodles with sauce and serve. Bon appétit!

Nutrition: 194 Calories; 17.1g Fat; 7.6g Carbs; 2.5g Protein; 4.6g Fiber

Balkan-Style Stir-Fry

Prep Time: 25 minutes | **Serve:** 5

- 8 bell peppers, deveined and cut into strips
- 1 tomato, chopped
- 2 eggs
- 1 yellow onion, sliced
- 3 garlic cloves, halved

1. Heat 2 tablespoons of olive oil in a saucepan over medium-low flame. Sweat the onion for about 4 minutes or until tender and translucent.

2. Stir in the garlic and peppers and continue to sauté for 5 to 6 minutes. Fold in chopped tomato along with salt and black pepper.

3.Stir fry for a further 7 minutes. Stir in the eggs and continue to cook for 4 to 5 minutes longer. Serve immediately.

Nutrition: 114 Calories; 7.6g Fat; 6g Carbs; 3.4g Protein; 1.5g Fiber

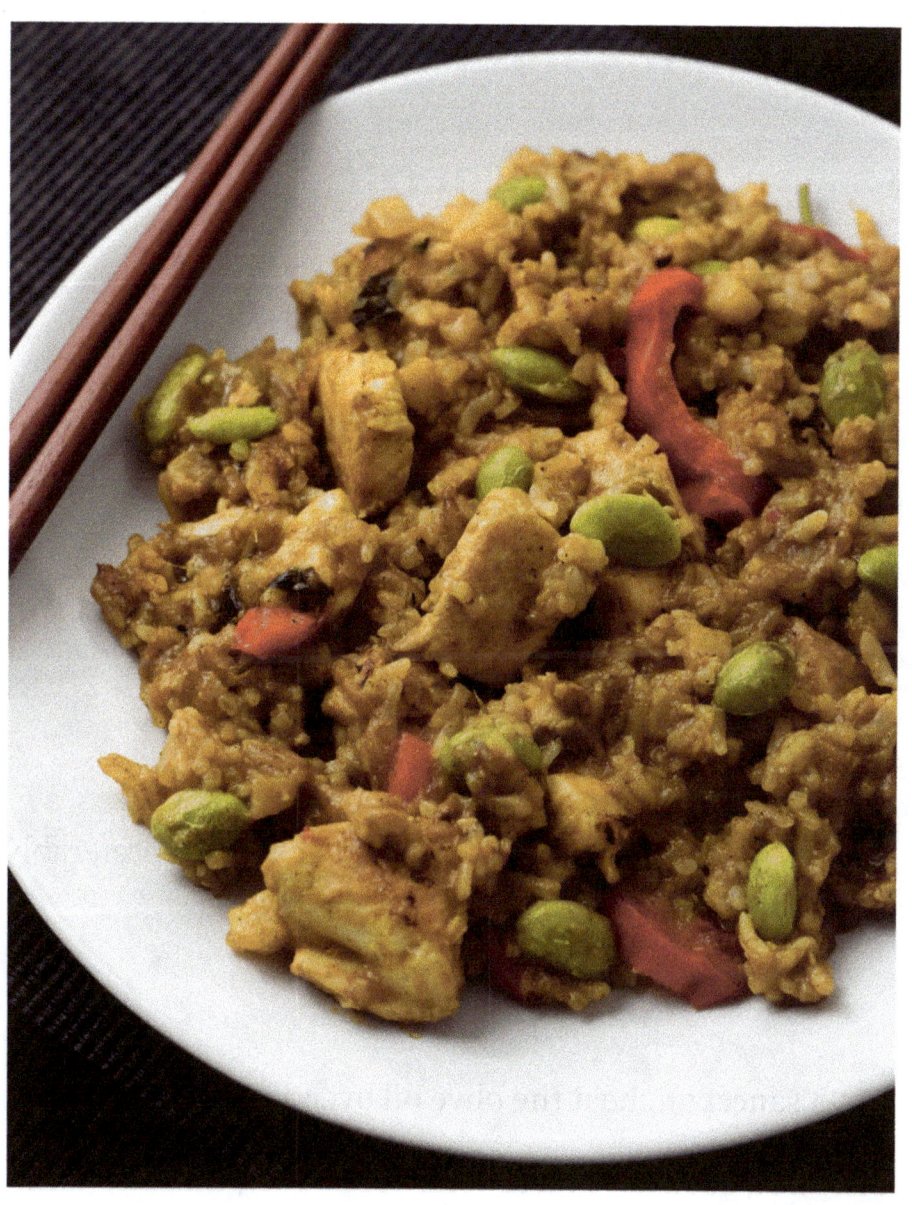

Italian Zoodles with Romano Cheese

Prep Time: 15 minutes | **Serve:** 3

- 1 ½ tablespoons olive oil
- 3 cups button mushrooms, chopped
- 1 cup tomato sauce with garlic and herbs
- 1 pound zucchini, spiralized
- 1/3 cup Pecorino Romano cheese, preferably freshly grated

1. In a saucepan, heat the olive oil over a moderate heat. Once hot, cook the mushrooms for about 4 minutes until they have softened.

2.Stir in the tomato sauce and zucchini, bringing to a boil.

3.Immediately reduce temperature to simmer. Continue to cook, partially covered, for about 7 minutes or until cooked through. Season with salt and black pepper.

4.Top with Pecorino Romano cheese and serve. Bon appétit!

Nutrition: 160 Calories; 10.6g Fat; 7.4g Carbs; 10g Protein; 3.4g Fiber

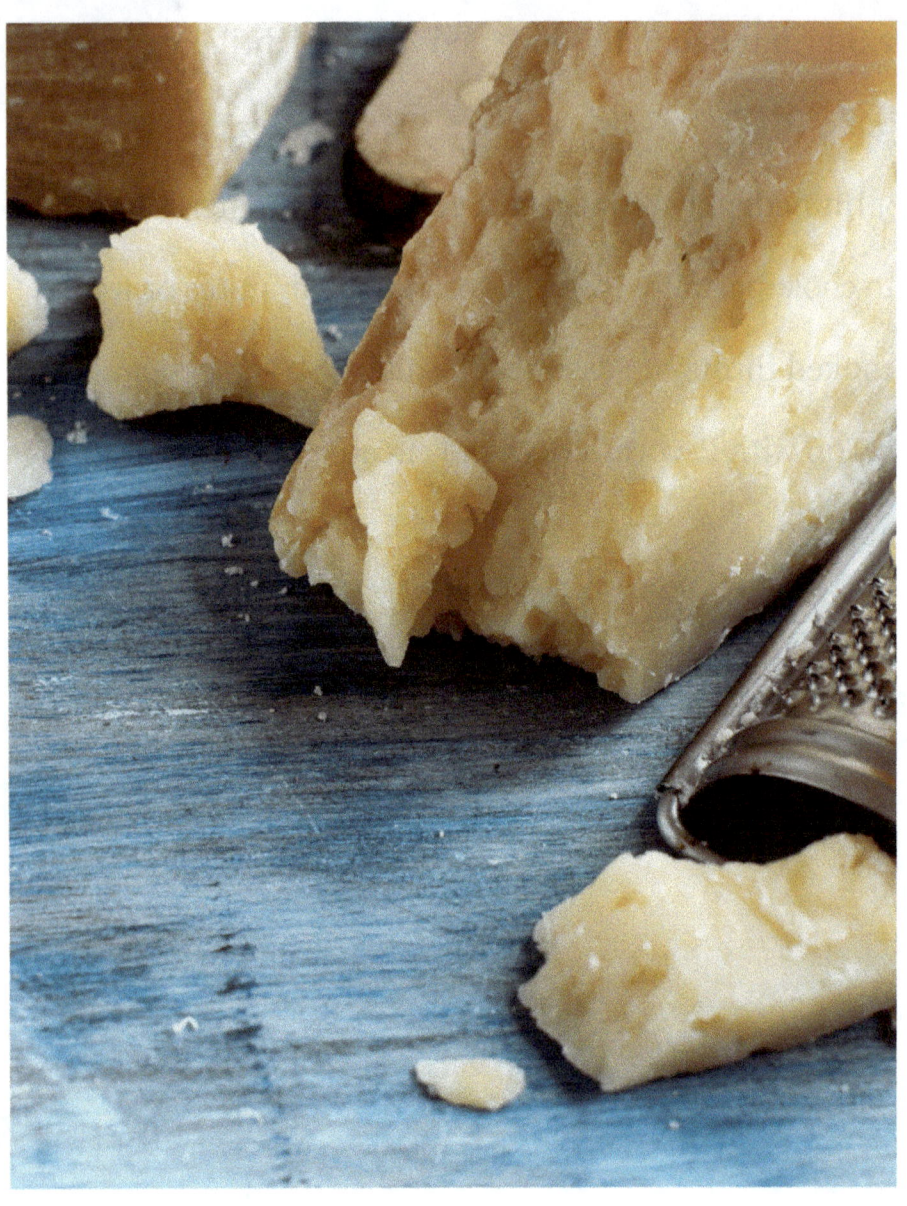

www.ingramcontent.com/pod-product-compliance
Lightning Source LLC
Chambersburg PA
CBHW070725030426
42336CB00013B/1920